Real World Medicine

Real World Medicine

WHAT YOUR ATTENDING DIDN'T TELL YOU AND YOUR PROFESSOR DIDN'T KNOW

Stephanie E. Freeman, MD, MBA

purposely
created
PUBLISHING

REAL WORLD MEDICINE

Published by Purposely Created Publishing Group™

Copyright © 2017 Stephanie E. Freeman

Printed in the United States of America

ISBN: 978-1-945558-66-5

Special discounts are available on bulk quantity purchases by book clubs, associations, and special interest groups. For details email:
sales@publishyourgift.com
or call (888) 949-6228.

For information logon to:
www.PublishYourGift.com

Dedication

For my mom: my greatest teacher,
best friend, and biggest supporter.

Table of Contents

Introduction

The process of becoming a physician is extremely challenging. After undergraduate school, it takes a minimum of seven years to get through medical school, internships, residencies, and fellowships, which are all designed to ensure that physicians get the best training possible. Countless hours are spent studying, rounding on patients, taking calls, and taking a seemingly endless number of exams, however, many physicians have discovered that practicing medicine in the real world as an attending physician—not within the confines of a training program—has its unique set of challenges.

Many of the issues faced by young physicians just entering into the practice of medicine are common to all physicians, but many physicians are not trained to deal with these situations because their medical schools and post-graduate training programs offer little training in the nonclinical aspects of medical practice. I have been practicing medicine as a critical care physician for 10 years. The vast majority of that time has been spent working as a locum tenens physician. Throughout my career as a locums physician, I have worked in many hospitals and have met numerous attending physicians, medical residents, and medical students. I am always astonished at the disconnect between what we as physicians are taught during our medical training and what we actually have to know as physicians in the real world.

I wrote this book to help bridge that gap. *Real World Medicine: What Your Attending Didn't Tell You and Your Professor Didn't Know* provides practical advice on how to have a successful career in medicine. This book discusses many of the issues faced by physicians and offers solid strategies on how to navigate the complex legal, financial, and political aspects of practicing medicine that will help you avoid the common mistakes many physicians make.

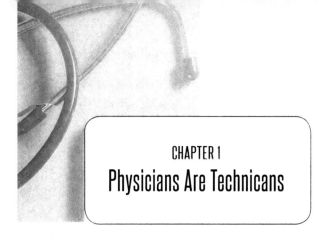

CHAPTER 1
Physicians Are Technicans

Medicine is an art. Medicine is a science. Medicine is also a business. The fact that medicine is a business catches a lot of physicians off guard. Medical practices, hospitals, nursing homes, and healthcare systems must all make money in order to continue to provide medical services for patients. In the business of medicine, physicians are unfortunately seen as and treated as technicians. We are expected to do the work but have no input in how things are actually run. Hospitals are run by MBAs, not MDs. Most hospital CEOs have no medical training and have never taken care of patients. They often have no idea what it takes to care for a patient. In fact, I once had a CEO tell me that my job as a critical care physician running a 28-bed ICU could never be as stressful as his job as a CEO. The fact that I make life-and-death decisions multiple times every single day meant absolutely nothing to this CEO, who spends his days in meetings.

Decisions regarding the systems, operations, structure, and finances of healthcare organizations are made by administrators. More often than not, physicians have no input into these decisions. However, physicians generate all the revenue for these organizations. Our contribution to these organizations is often minimized to how many patients we see and how much we bill for our patient encounters. Thus, many times, our roles are diminished to that of a technician. Again, we do the work but get no say in how things are run.

Along those lines, here is the harsh reality regarding the business of medicine. First of all, if you do not make money for your organization, you may be fired. Businesses must be profitable in order to remain in business. The biggest expense in any business is the employees. If it costs more money to employ you than you generate in revenue, then your job is in jeopardy.

In order to prevent this from happening, you need to do

several things. First of all, you must know how much money you are costing the organization. This includes things like your salary, sign-on bonuses, relocation expenses, loan repayment, benefits package, and malpractice insurance. In addition to that, you must know how much money you are making for your institution. In order to determine this, you need to know the appropriate current procedural terminology (CPT) code for your services, the appropriate ICD-10 code for the diagnoses, and the RVU for each service and procedure you perform. RVU stands for relative value unit. It is a component of the Center for Medicare and Medicaid's (CMS) Resource Based Relative Value Scale, which is a system used to determine how much will be paid by insurance companies and organizations for physician services. The CMS physician fee schedule can be found online at the CMS website and will give the RVUs and the dollar amount corresponding to the CPT code.

With this information, you can determine how many RVUs you need to generate in order to cover your salary. You can also figure out how many patients you need to see daily, or how many of a certain type of procedure you need to do in order to generate revenue and to be profitable. Meet with your organization's billing and coding department so you can get more information about this as it pertains specifically to your organization. They will certainly appreciate your interest, as many physicians have no interest in finances and are clueless as it pertains to them. Having a good understanding of billing and coding allows you to ensure that you and your organization are getting adequately compensated for the work that you do. Errors in billing and coding are quite costly and can negatively impact the finances of the physician and the organization.

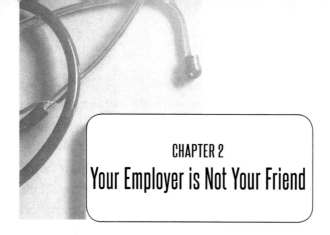

CHAPTER 2
Your Employer is Not Your Friend

Healthcare organizations exist to provide a service and to make money in the process. Period. When they hire you, they hire you to provide a service that they can profit from. The employer–employee relationship is a business transaction in which you are paid money in exchange for the services you provide your employer. Regardless of how nice they appear and how great a place it may be to work, always keep in mind that your employer places the good of the business/institution/organization above your individual needs as an employee. Their interests are not necessarily in your best interest.

Many physicians have been recruited to work for organizations that were eager to hire them for their services, only to be fired a few months later when the organization suffered a financial loss and needed to downsize its workforce. Therefore, it is imperative that you keep abreast of everything that is going on in your organization. Be aware of the financial status of your organization. Many organizations release quarterly reports that provide valuable information regarding the health of the company. Keep up with changes in leadership, ownership of the company, and any external forces that can impact the company.

Physician Employment Contracts

Your employment contract is written to protect the interests of your employer. Therefore, they typically insert certain things in physician contracts that may not be found in other employment contracts.

As a result, there are several items that physicians must pay particular attention to pertaining to their employment contracts. The first one is to know who your contract is with. Is it with a hospital or is it with a physician group or corporation that has a contract with the hospital? Is it with the healthcare organization that owns the hospital, office, clinic, etc.? For example, you are a hospitalist who has been recruited to work at Acme Hospital. Are you going to be an employee of the hospital or are you going to be an employee of the XYZ Hospitalist Group that provides hospitalist services for Acme Hospital? Furthermore, if XYZ Hospitalist Group is a national company, they may be doing business in your particular state under another name due to state legal requirements. XYZ Hospitalist Group is based in Florida, but in Texas, they operate as ABC Hospitalist Group. Be aware of whose name is on the contract so that you will know who your contract is actually with. Therefore, if a legal issue arises, you will know who to deal with and how to contact them.

Secondly, be sure the contract describes the job in detail and lists the job duties, work hours, work schedule, on-call schedule, and work location. Furthermore, the compensation terms should be clearly delineated in the contract. The compensation, bonuses, benefits, and malpractice insurance all need to be clearly stated. The contract needs to describe in detail how you will be paid. Is it in the form of a salary or is it based on production according to the RVUs generated? If production based, what is the formula used to determine the productivity and the dollar amount paid? Is there a "claw back" provision that states if you are paid a certain amount and do not produce that amount, you have to pay back that extra amount you were paid? If your contract states you are paid hourly per shift, do you get paid extra if you stay late? If your contract states you work a set number of shifts each month, do you get paid for the additional shifts you work? If so, at what rate?

I know of a group of hospitalists who were not paid for working additional shifts even though their contract specified that they would be. They had to threaten to sue the hospital in order to get their back pay. I also know physicians who had to pay back money to their employers after failing to meet the productivity targets set forth in their contracts. In order to avoid these issues, you need to have a good understanding of your contract. Read the contract thoroughly and have it reviewed in detail by an attorney who is an expert in physician employment contracts.

If your compensation is salary plus production bonuses, be sure to know what your base salary is and how your production bonuses will be determined. Also, the contract needs to specify when bonuses will be paid. Some compensation models start off as fully salaried and then transition to production based over a period of years. If this is the case, your contract must specify over which period of time this transition will occur and how your productivity will be determined.

You must also pay attention to the termination clause. Most physician contracts are three years. Grounds for early termination of the contract can be "for cause" or "without cause." The employer can terminate a physician's contract immediately for cause for events including loss of medical license, loss of hospital privileges, commission of a crime, misconduct, and exclusion from third-party payers. Without-cause termination can be initiated by either the employee or employer, and this usually requires a 30-, 60-, or 90-day notice. If the employer terminates the contract without cause and has the employee cease working on the day of termination, the employer usually continues to pay the salary through length of the notice period. Depending on who initiates the termination and for what reason determines who will pay for malpractice tail coverage, among other things. Some contracts state that if a physician is terminated for cause or terminates the contract without cause, then the physician is responsible for paying for tail coverage for the malpractice insurance. Furthermore, the contract may also require that the physician pay back any sign-on bonuses, loan repayments, pre-employment stipends, recruitment fees, and moving expenses. I once resigned from a job after having worked there for nine months and was told by my employer that, based on the terms of the contract, I had to repay the $20,000 sign-on bonus and pay $7,000 for malpractice tail coverage.

Another major item included in physician contracts is the non-compete clause, also known as a restrictive covenant. As the name implies, these clauses are designed to keep the physicians from competing with their employer. This is included in physician contracts to prevent physicians from practicing medicine within a certain-mile radius of the organization for a specific period of time after the physician is no longer employed by the organization. For example, a physician may be prohibited from practicing medicine within a 25-mile radius of their employer for a length of two years. Depending on the size of the practice location, that 25-mile restrictive covenant may encompass such a broad area that the physician may be forced to relocate to another area in order to find work. On the other hand, in larger cities, the restrictive covenant may be 2.5, 5, or 10 miles. A physician may easily find another job in a city that does not violate her restrictive covenant.

Another issue regarding employment contracts that physicians must consider is their intellectual property. Many organizations are including clauses in their employment contracts that claim ownership of the physician's intellectual property created while the physician is employed with that organization. A typical clause may read as such: "Any work of authorship or invention created by an employee during the scope of his or her employment with XYZ Organization shall be considered the property of XYZ Organization, including any patent, trademark, copyright, trade secret, or other intellectual property right in such work of authorship or invention." This means that your employer can claim ownership of any of the intellectual property you create during your employment with them. Let's say you write a bestselling novel during the time you are not at work. If your contract has a clause claiming ownership of your intellectual property, then your employer will be entitled to the ownership of your novel and the monies the novel generates.

Furthermore, physicians must determine whether their employment contract allows them to provide any professional services outside of their work for their employer. They must make sure the employment contract does not prohibit activities such as moonlighting, consulting, providing expert witness, speaking, etc. If moonlighting is allowed, it must be specified whether the employer's malpractice policy will cover it, or whether a separate policy covering the moonlighting activities must be obtained. If outside professional activities are allowed, the contract must specify whether the income generated from such activities belongs to the physician or the employer.

Negotiating Skills

Physicians are taught many things throughout the course of their training. However, we are not taught how to negotiate. As a result, many physicians are uncomfortable talking about money and asking for more money. Male physicians are paid more than female physicians, and white physicians are paid more than black physicians. Therefore, it is crucial that every physician know how to negotiate in order to make sure she is getting paid what she is worth.

The first step in negotiating is to find out what other physicians are getting paid. Although discussing salaries with your coworkers may be considered taboo, the easiest way to find out what other physicians are making is to ask them. Ask physicians in your specialty about their salary and benefits. Talk to physicians locally and in other parts of the country. Next, read the *Medscape Physician Compensation Report* and the *MGMA Physician Compensation Report*. These reports contain important information about physician salaries nationwide. Thirdly, talk to job recruiters. They have firsthand knowledge of what jobs are paying. Finally, if you are renegotiating a contract, don't be afraid to start an actual job search. Go on interviews and talk with other potential employers. You can use this information as leverage in your negotiations with your current employer.

Furthermore, you must determine what value you add to the company. How much money do you generate for your employer? How productive are you? How many RVUs do you generate? If you are just negotiating an initial contract, you can estimate these numbers based on the expected workload. For example, if your potential employer tells you that you will see an average of 25 patients each day in an outpatient practice, you can estimate the number of RVUs you will generate and base your contract negotiations around that. Employers already have this data and this is what they are basing their offer on. You must have this same information so that you can challenge their assumptions and feel comfortable rejecting the first contract they offer you, if it's not what you know you should be getting or think you deserve.

Another thing that you must do before you start negotiating your contract is to determine exactly what you want. Do you have a particular salary in mind? What benefits do you want? How much PTO? Vacation? Sick leave? Maternity leave? Administrative time? Do you want to have Fridays off? Determine exactly what you want so you can be sure to ask for it. You can't just assume that employers know what you want and will automatically offer it. By specifically asking for what you want, you increase your chances of getting it.

Lastly, consider the alternatives. What are you willing to do if your employer/future employer says no? A no today does not mean no tomorrow. If they do not agree to your request, ask your employer what must be done so that you can get your request granted at a later date. If they don't agree to all of your terms, get them to agree on some of your terms. Negotiation does not have to be an "all-or-nothing" game. If the negatives of staying at your job outweigh the positives, it may be time to leave. Be willing to walk away.

As you can see, physician employment contracts are extremely complex and are written to protect the interests of the employer. As a physician, you must assemble a team of experts who will work on your behalf to protect your interests. You need an attorney, a certified professional accountant, and a financial planner, all of whom are experts in medical, legal, and financial issues as they pertain to physicians. Have all of your contracts reviewed by your attorney and discuss your contract in detail with him or her. It is imperative that you understand every single word of your contract. Failure to do so may not only cost you time and money but could also jeopardize your medical career.

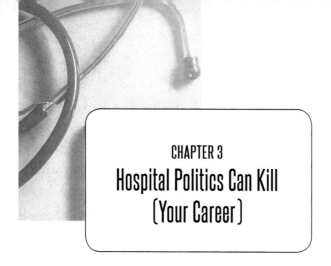

CHAPTER 3
Hospital Politics Can Kill (Your Career)

"It's not what you know, it's who you know." This old statement also rings true in the clinical setting. Your skills as a physician will only take you so far. Your interpersonal skills and relationships with others will determine your success within an organization, and having a good rapport with the "higher-ups" makes it more likely they will help you when an issue arises.

All too often, physicians work with their heads buried in the sand, so to speak. We are so busy seeing patients that we often do not know who the major decision makers are. As a result, when something happens, we don't know who to turn to. It is imperative that you know all the members of the administration: the chief executive officer (CEO), chief medical officer (CMO), chief nursing officer (CNO), and chief operating officer (COO). In addition, make it a point to know all of the directors and managers in the hospital units and in the outpatient facilities in which you will be working. If you are employed by a physician group, know who the partners are. If you are employed by a physician employment company, you must know your local medical director, regional medical director, CMO, and CEO of the organization.

Physicians must know how to navigate political relationships within several arenas. Not only must you get along with the physicians and administrators in your group, but you must get along well with the physicians, nurses, managers, and administrators in every hospital and every facility in which you work. For example, your group may love you, but you may not be well liked at a particular hospital. Take Dr. X. Dr. X is an anesthesiologist who is well liked by her fellow anesthesiologists. However, Dr. X is not well liked at ACME surgical center, and the nurses have complained to Dr. X's employers. As a result, Dr. X's employer had to reassign Dr. X to another surgical center.

Along with forming positive relationships with everyone, you must know who the "untouchables" are. By that I mean you must know who the physicians are who have the most power and influence, and who can get away with essentially anything. Every facility has them, and you must know who they are. These are the physicians who, regardless of their clinical performance and professional behavior, are never sanctioned or admonished by administration. Many of these physicians have been at these organizations for decades, and they may be the largest revenue generators of the organizations. You must take care not to cross these physicians. Even if you are right in a particular instance, they may retaliate against you. Due to their influence and power in that institution, you may end up on the losing end of that battle. That is why having a good rapport with the administrators in your organization is essential—so that they can at least be receptive to what you have to say regarding the matter.

There are several committees that exist in hospitals that you must be aware of in order to know how the hospital operates in terms of the medical staff:

- The **medical executive committee (MEC)** is the governance committee of the medical staff. Its duty is to implement policies, procedures, and rules as they pertain to the medical staff.

- The **peer review committee** is made up of physicians. Its role is to review the work of a physician to see whether the standard of care has been rendered.

- The **credentialing committee** does just what its name implies: grants the appropriate credentials to physicians.

- The **quality assurance committee** is concerned with performance improvement and patient safety, among other things.

Every healthcare organization has its own unique culture. They all have one thing they value over everything else. You must find out what that one thing is. Some organizations pride themselves on their family-like atmosphere. Other organizations value strategic growth. Others pride themselves on their safety and quality. You must find out what the organization's culture is and whether or not you fit into it. If you are a person who likes being a part of fast-growing, innovative organizations, then working for an organization that focuses on everybody liking everybody else and having a "family-like" atmosphere, may not be right for you. When interviewing with an organization, ask specifically what the organization values. They will say things like "growth," " innovation," " research," " family-like atmosphere," "superior patient care," etc. If you have any doubts that you will fit into an organization, you probably won't, and you should look for another job.

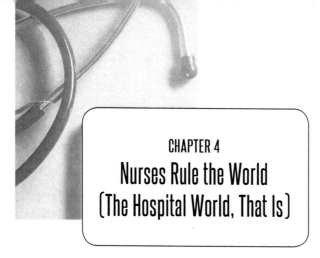

CHAPTER 4
Nurses Rule the World
(The Hospital World, That Is)

Nurses run the hospital. The nursing staff is the most powerful and influential body in the hospital. There is an old saying: "Nurses can make or break you." I used to doubt this statement early in my career, until I saw this happen first hand and experienced this personally. The nurses always have the ear of the administration. The bedside nurse reports to the charge nurse. The charge nurse reports to the unit director. The unit director reports to the CNO. The CNO reports to the CEO. So any issue a nurse has with a physician is much more likely to be brought to the attention of administration than vice versa. Physicians have a chain of command that starts with the director of the department and then proceeds to the CMO and then the CEO. However, in my experience, nurses are more likely to report an issue with a physician than physicians are to report an issue with a nurse.

As a result of this, it is imperative that you get along with the nursing staff. Rule number one: be nice to them. This should be common sense; however, some physicians are not very nice to nurses and, as a result, nurses don't like working with them. As the old saying goes, "You catch more flies with honey than you do with vinegar." Remember, the nurse is at the patients' bedsides 8 to 12 hours each day. He or she is your eyes and ears as it pertains to the patient. Listen to your nurse. Respect what the nurse has to say. Be sure to value their input.

Be aware that nothing you ever say to a nurse is truly "off the record." Comments that you make casually regarding a patient or the treatment plan can wind up in the patient's record in the nursing notes. Nurses have a lot of freedom regarding what they choose to document. This has happened to me before. Once, a nurse notified me that a patient had arrived to the ICU. The patient was hemodynamically stable and nothing needed to be done immediately for the patient. I told her that I would see the patient once

I returned from lunch. Instead of the nurse documenting "the patient has arrived to the unit, Dr. Freeman aware," the nurse documented, "Dr. Freeman notified that patient has arrived. She stated that she will see the patient when she returns from lunch."

I did not expect the fact that I was taking a well-deserved lunch break to end up in the patient's medical record, as it had nothing to do with the care of the patient. This taught me a very important lesson. I learned that nurses are paying close attention to everything physicians do and say. As a result, we always have to be "on." We can never have a bad day. We can never lose our cool or express frustration about a situation or event. Our actions, behavior, and speech in regard to patient care can end up in the patient record.

Never ever make disparaging comments about the patient. Never ever express frustration at the nurse about a situation. Even if the nurse calls you at 2:15 a.m. about a seemingly inconsequential lab value, don't ever say, "Well, what do you want me to do about that?" Trust me, the nurse will document your statement, and if there is ever an issue with the patient, since your statement is in the record, you will have to answer for it. Along those lines, always read the nurses notes to make sure the information is accurate.

Nurses are a tight-knit group of people. They gossip a lot about each other and about other physicians. Never tell a nurse anything that you don't want the whole hospital to eventually know. Keep your interactions with the nurses and other staff members polite and pleasant. Avoid discussing sensitive topics such as politics, religion, money, etc. It is very difficult to overcome the dislike of the nursing staff. Their dislike of you can cost you your job. I was once on a locums assignment at a hospital in West Virginia. An ICU nurse decided that she did not like me. She told the administration that she would quit if they did not terminate my locums assignment. I was well liked by the other ICU nurses, however, because this particular nurse was a clinical instructor of nursing, she was more valuable to the organization than I was as a critical care physician. The hospital felt that they could replace me more easily than they could replace her; therefore, they terminated my assignment. Remember, nurses complain, and they have the ear of the administration. If your employer or hospital administration gets enough complaints about you from the nursing staff, whether substantiated or not, they will fire you.

On the other hand, if the nursing staff likes you, they will advocate for you, and it may end up advancing your career. There was one particular instance where I had done some locums work at a hospital on several occasions. I got along really well with the nursing staff and really enjoyed working with them. After a few months of not working at that hospital, the medical director called me and asked me to return. He stated that the nurses had requested that he bring me back to work there.

Getting along with the nursing staff everywhere you work is mandatory if you want a pleasant work environment. This is not to say that you must accept shoddy work or bad behavior on their part, but you must treat them with professional courtesy and respect. You don't have to be friends with the nurses, but you must be friendly toward the nurses.

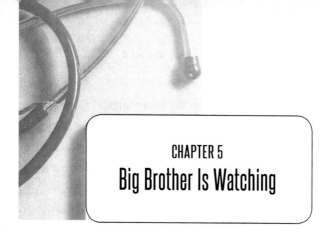

CHAPTER 5
Big Brother Is Watching

Physicians are constantly being watched. Our behavior is being monitored by everyone, from the general public, patients, staff, administration, private insurance companies, the federal government, and state medical boards. Everybody is watching us. This is not to instill paranoia but to bring awareness to the various ways in which physicians are monitored and our behavior is tracked.

The administration of your hospital and your employer are keeping tabs on your productivity and the quality of care you provide. Physicians are constantly being economically credentialed, so to speak. By this I mean that administrators are always looking at how much money you are making the organization or costing the organization. They want to know the (monetary) value you add. Administrators want to know how many patients you see, how many patients you admit to the hospital, what procedures you perform, how many RVUs you generate, the average length of stay for your patients, the morbidity and mortality of your patients, and the case mix of your patients. Physicians must also meet certain performance measures. Medicare and Medicaid, along with private insurance companies, provide financial incentives and penalties for meeting or failing to meet certain standards. Therefore, you need to find out what metrics are being measured and how your performance measures up.

The general public holds physicians in high esteem and places a lot of trust in us. As a result, the general public, our patients, and the state medical boards hold physicians to a high standard of ethics and behavior. Often, physicians fail to realize that our behavior outside the hospital or medical office can place our careers in jeopardy. Being convicted of a crime, even if that action does not involve patient care, can place the physician at risk of losing her medical license. For example, some physicians have been convicted of tax evasion and have lost their license as a result. Even if a criminal conviction does not result in the loss of a medical license, it could result in the loss of employment and the loss of the ability to participate in all federal healthcare programs such as Medicare and Medicaid.

In addition to being convicted of a crime, there are several other reasons a physician may lose his license to practice medicine. These include inappropriate prescribing of controlled substances, failure to provide standard of care, inappropriate relationships with patients, misconduct, negligence, substance abuse, and medical conditions that impair a physician's ability to practice medicine. Furthermore, there are certain events that must be reported to the medical board, and failure to do so may result in a loss of license. I recommend that you are very familiar with the rules of your state medical board.

In addition to the state medical boards, the National Practitioner Data Bank (NPDB) is a national organization that compiles a list of adverse events and formal complaints lodged against physicians. The NPDB collects information and reports on medical malpractice payments, licensure actions, adverse actions against clinical privileges, poor accreditation performance, sanctions by peer review committees, healthcare-related criminal convictions or civil judgments, and exclusions from participation in state or federal health programs. State medical boards and the NPDB are queried by all employers, hospitals, insurance companies, and any other healthcare organization regarding individual physicians.

Disruptive physician behavior can also be reported to the state medical board and the NPDB. Disruptive physician behavior includes belittling or berating statements, use of profanity, offensive jokes, sexual harassment, racial insensitivity, physical threats, physical contact, failure to return phone calls or pages, throwing things, etc. Being labeled a "disruptive physician" can result in the termination of employment, loss of hospital privileges, expulsion from insurance plans, investigations by the state medical board, and being reported to the NPDB.

If a physician engages in any of these behaviors, he or she deserves to be labeled as disruptive" and to face the consequences. However, sometimes a physician who does not exhibit this type of behavior can be labeled as such simply because he or she is not liked by some people in the organization. Labeling a physician as disruptive may be used as a tactic of the hospital administration and employers to retaliate against a physician they do not like. Often, they threaten to report the physician to the medical board for "disruptive" behavior as a way to silence the physician or retaliate against them. I once worked for a hospital that threatened to report me to the medical board for being a disruptive physician simply because I complained to the administration about the excessive workload and the unsafe work conditions. Therefore, not only must physicians be on their best behavior at all times, but they must take any verbal or written threat to label them as disruptive very seriously and seek legal counsel.

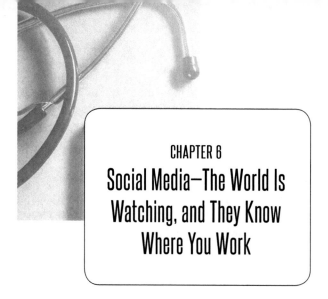

CHAPTER 6

Social Media—The World Is Watching, and They Know Where You Work

Social media has changed the way the world communicates. As the use of social media expands, its role in healthcare is expanding and changing as well. As a result, physicians must be especially careful when using social media. Physicians must ensure that all methods of communicating with patients are compliant with HIPPA. Emailing and videoconferencing with patients must be done on a secure network that meets the specifications of both HIPPA and HITECH. Text messaging to patients and to other physicians regarding patient care must be avoided unless it is ensured that the network is secured. Posts to social media websites regarding patient care must be done with care as to not violate that patient's privacy. Written consent must be obtained if personal information about the patient is shared. If written consent is not obtained, care must be taken and the post written in such a way that the patient's identity cannot be recognized.

Some experts recommend not "friending" patients on your social media account, or, if you do so, to establish a professional social media account in addition to your personal social media account. Avoid posting things on your social media accounts that show you in an unprofessional light. For example, avoid showing pictures of you being intoxicated or in other compromising positions. This raises questions about your professional conduct and your skills as a physician. In addition to that, avoid offensive posts on your social media accounts. Increasingly, healthcare professionals, including physicians, are losing their jobs as a result of offensive social media posts.

Conclusion

After years of training, physicians are so excited about the chance to practice medicine in the real world. We want the opportunity to put our training to good use and to provide the best care that we can for our patients. However, there are many situations, as discussed in this book, that can derail or destroy a physician's career. These are things that were not taught to us during our training. Therefore, physicians must understand the business of medicine and what our roles are.

We must be savvy when it comes to negotiating contracts, not only to ensure that we are paid what we are worth, but to ensure that we don't enter into contracts with unreasonable stipulations. We must know how to navigate the world of hospital politics and learn how to develop professional relationships with the staff, nurses, and administrators. Furthermore, we must be aware of the various regulatory agencies and how they can affect our career. Finally, we must keep up with the ever-changing world of social media and learn how to engage in such a way that is beneficial to our patients while protecting their privacy.

With some planning and expert guidance, physicians can navigate these areas with ease and will be able to enjoy many satisfying years in the field of medicine.

About the Author

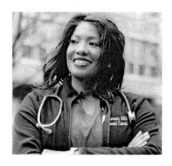

Stephanie E. Freeman, MD, MBA, is a board-certified critical care physician, bestselling author of *Locum Tenens: Your Questions Answered*, speaker, and consultant. Known as the Job Doctor, Dr. Stephanie's mission is to help physicians regain control of their lives by finding alternative jobs and careers in medicine so they can practice medicine on their own terms. As the founder and chief medical advisor of DrStephanieICU.com, she consistently meets with physicians individually and in groups to discuss ways they can get "unstuck" in their careers and real-world career strategies to help physicians think outside the box.

Dr. Stephanie earned her medical degree from the University of Alabama School of Medicine, and completed her internal medicine residency at Wake Forest University Baptist Medical Center and her critical care fellowship at the University of Pittsburgh Medical Center. Dr. Stephanie also completed a geriatrics fellowship at Wake Forest University Baptist Medical Center and obtained her masters of business administration at Auburn University.

In her spare time, Dr. Stephanie enjoys reading and indoor cycling. She currently resides in Houston, Texas.

To connect, visit her website at www.drstephanieicu.com.

CREATING DISTINCTIVE BOOKS
WITH INTENTIONAL RESULTS

We're a collaborative group of creative masterminds
with a mission to produce high-quality books to position
you for monumental success in the marketplace.

Our professional team of writers, editors, designers,
and marketing strategists work closely together to ensure
that every detail of your book is a clear representation
of the message in your writing.

Want to know more?
Write to us at info@publishyourgift.com
or call (888) 949-6228

Discover great books, exclusive offers, and more at
www.PublishYourGift.com

Connect with us on social media

@publishyourgift

CPSIA information can be obtained
at www.ICGtesting.com
Printed in the USA
LVOW07s0503051017
551257LV00024B/203/P